MINDFUL HYPNOBIRTHING

Hypnosis and Mindfulness Practices for a Confident and Serene Birth

By: Lisa Freeman

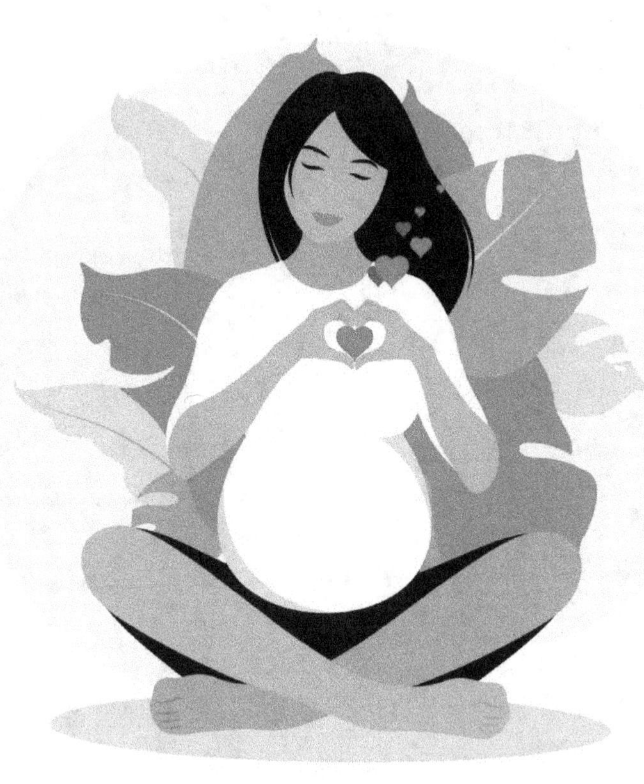

purview. There are no scenarios in which the publisher or the original author of this work can be in any fashion deemed liable for any hardship or damages that may befall them after undertaking information described herein.

Additionally, the information in the following pages is intended only for informational purposes and should thus be thought of as universal. As befitting its nature, it is presented without assurance regarding its prolonged validity or interim quality. Trademarks that are mentioned are done without written consent and can in no way be considered an endorsement from the trademark holder.

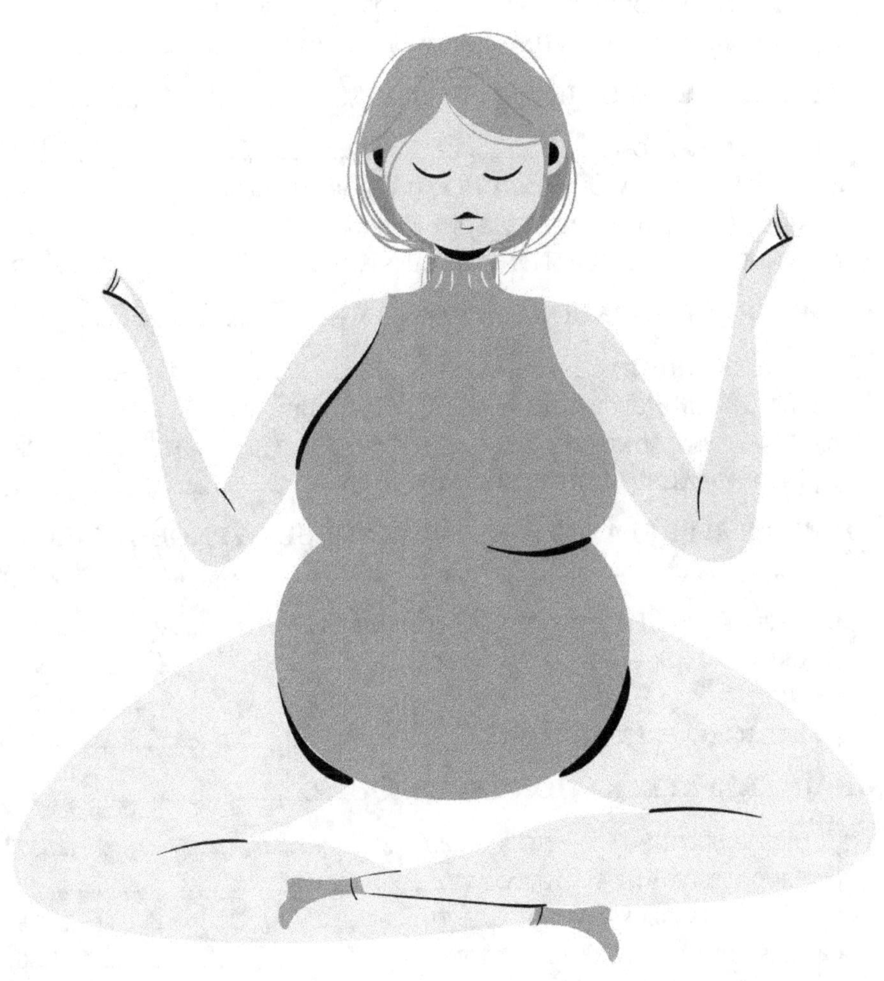

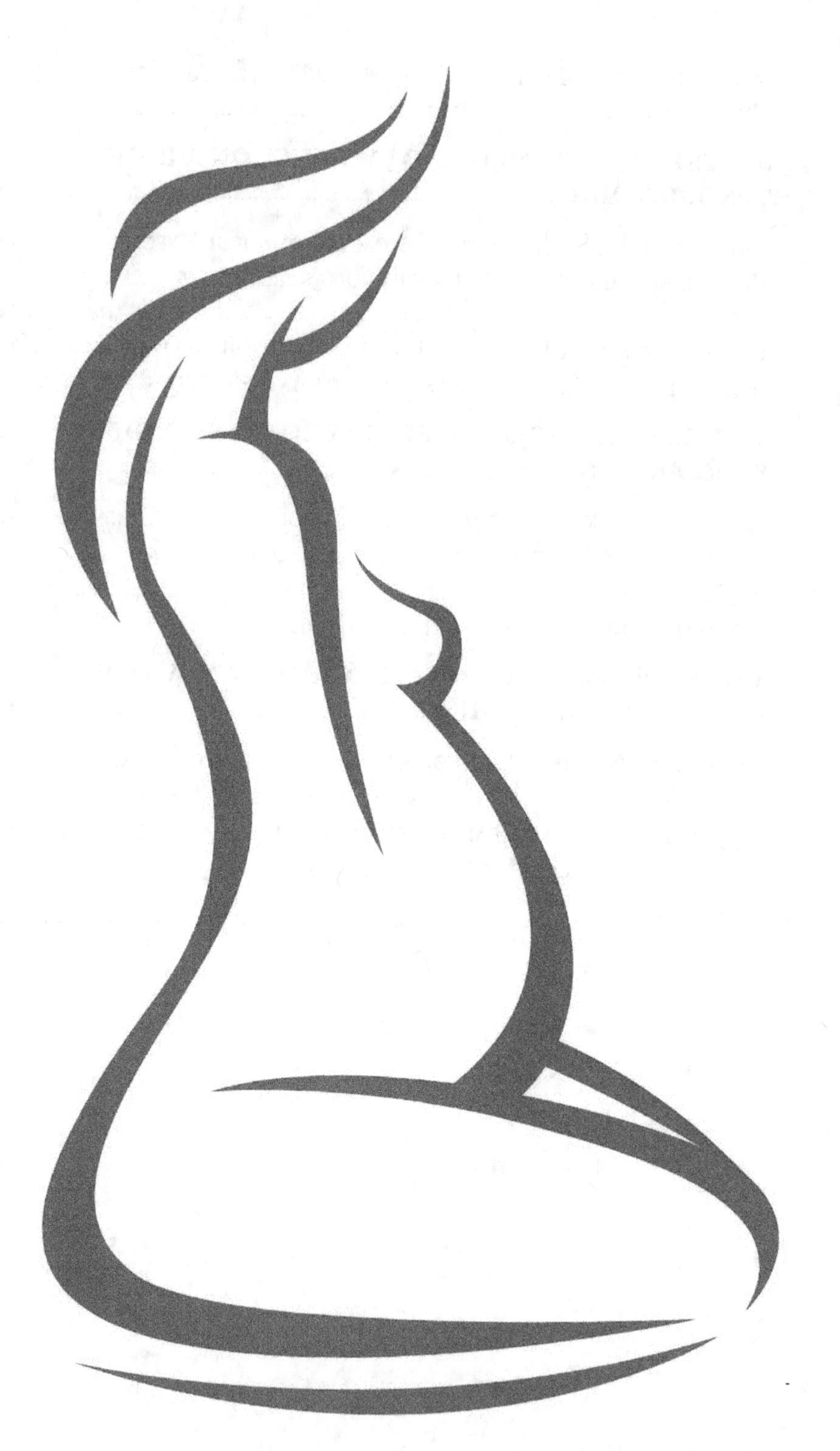

1.1 THE CONCEPT OF MINDFUL HYPNOBIRTHING

Mindful Hypnobirthing is a holistic approach to childbirth that combines mindfulness and hypnosis techniques to promote a calm and confident birthing experience. It emphasizes the power of the mind-body connection and aims to empower expectant mothers to have a positive and empowering birth journey. This chapter provides an overview of the concept of Mindful Hypnobirthing, its origins, and the principles it is based on. Mindful Hypnobirthing draws inspiration from various practices, including hypnotherapy, mindfulness meditation, and positive psychology. It recognizes that childbirth can be a transformative and natural process and seeks to shift the perception of birth from a medical event to a profound and empowering life experience. By integrating mindfulness and hypnosis, Mindful Hypnobirthing enables women to tap into their inner resources, reduce fear and anxiety, and enhance their ability to navigate the birthing process.

1.2 BENEFITS OF MINDFULNESS AND HYPNOSIS DURING BIRTH

The incorporation of mindfulness and hypnosis techniques during childbirth offers numerous benefits for both the mother and the baby. By practicing mindfulness, expectant mothers develop the ability to be fully present in the moment, allowing them to connect with their bodies, acknowledge their sensations, and embrace the birthing process without judgment or resistance. This cultivates a sense of inner calm and relaxation, reducing stress and fear associated with childbirth. Hypnosis, on the other hand, is a state of focused attention and heightened suggestibility, which can be utilized to create positive changes in perception, behavior, and physical sensations. During childbirth, hypnosis can help women enter a deep state of relaxation, manage pain effectively, and facilitate a smoother labor experience. It can also promote the release of endorphins, the body's natural pain-relieving hormones, and reduce the need for pharmacological interventions.

Furthermore, research suggests that the use of mindfulness and hypnosis techniques during birth may contribute to shorter labor duration, fewer medical interventions, decreased rates of cesarean sections, and improved maternal satisfaction with the birthing process. Additionally, babies born to mothers who practiced Mindful Hypnobirthing may experience a calmer transition into the world, exhibit higher Apgar scores, and have improved bonding and breastfeeding outcomes.

1.3 UNDERSTANDING THE MIND-BODY CONNECTION

The mind-body connection plays a crucial role in childbirth, and understanding its dynamics is fundamental to Mindful Hypnobirthing. The mind and body are intricately linked, with thoughts, emotions, and beliefs exerting a profound influence on physical experiences. When it comes to childbirth, fear, stress, and anxiety can trigger the release of stress hormones, leading to increased muscle tension, reduced blood flow, and a heightened perception of pain.

In contrast, cultivating a positive mindset, relaxation, and a sense of trust in the birthing process can promote the release of endorphins and oxytocin, hormones that support relaxation, pain relief, and the progression of labor. By acknowledging and addressing any fears or negative beliefs surrounding birth, expectant mothers can create a more favorable environment for a calm and confident birthing experience.

Mindful Hypnobirthing recognizes the power of thoughts, emotions, and language in shaping the birth experience. It encourages expectant mothers to reframe their beliefs about childbirth, replacing fear and doubt with confidence and trust in their bodies' innate wisdom. Through mindfulness and hypnosis techniques, women can cultivate a positive and empowering mindset, establish a deeper connection with their bodies, and enhance their ability to navigate the birthing process with grace and resilience. The introduction to Mindful Hypnobirthing provides a comprehensive overview of the concept, emphasizing the integration of mindfulness and hypnosis techniques to achieve a calm and confident birth. It highlights the benefits of incorporating these practices, including reduced stress, enhanced pain management, and improved birth outcomes. Understanding the mind-body connection is fundamental to Mindful Hypnobirthing, as it allows expectant mothers to harness the power of their thoughts and emotions, fostering a positive and empowering birthing experience

2.1 WHAT IS HYPNOSIS?

Hypnosis is a state of focused attention and heightened suggestibility that allows individuals to access their subconscious mind and make positive changes in perception, behavior, and physical sensations. Contrary to popular belief, hypnosis is not a state of unconsciousness or mind control. Instead, it is a natural and relaxed state of consciousness that we often experience in our daily lives, such as when we become deeply absorbed in a book or lose track of time while engaged in an enjoyable activity. During hypnosis, individuals enter a state of deep relaxation and focused concentration. This relaxed state allows access to the subconscious mind, which is responsible for our automatic thoughts, emotions, and behaviors. By bypassing the critical conscious mind, hypnosis enables individuals to explore and reshape deep-seated beliefs, overcome barriers, and tap into their inner resources.

2.2 HOW HYPNOSIS WORKS IN THE CONTEXT OF CHILDBIRTH

In the context of childbirth, hypnosis is utilized to create a state of deep relaxation, reduce fear and anxiety, and facilitate a smoother birthing process. Expectant mothers can learn self-hypnosis techniques or work with a trained hypnotherapist to enter a hypnotic state during labor and delivery. By inducing a relaxed and calm state, hypnosis can help manage pain, enhance the mind-body connection, and promote a positive birth experience. During childbirth, hypnosis can be used to reframe perceptions of pain, replacing them with sensations of pressure or comfort. By focusing on positive affirmations, visualizations, and relaxation techniques, women in a hypnotic state can alter their experience of labor, making it more manageable and less distressing. Hypnosis can also help women maintain a sense of control, confidence, and empowerment throughout the birthing process.

2.3 COMMON MISCONCEPTIONS ABOUT HYPNOSIS

There are several common misconceptions about hypnosis that can create apprehension or skepticism among individuals considering its use during childbirth. One misconception is that hypnosis involves surrendering control or being under the influence of the hypnotherapist. In reality, hypnosis is a collaborative process, and individuals maintain complete control over their thoughts, actions, and choices. Hypnosis is a tool that empowers individuals to access their own inner resources and make positive changes. Another misconception is that individuals can be stuck in a hypnotic state or unable to awaken from it. In truth, hypnosis is a naturally occurring state that individuals can enter and exit at will. Even in a deep state of hypnosis, individuals can regain full awareness and wake up if needed. Hypnosis is a safe and reversible process that respects an individual's autonomy and free will.

2.4 FINDING A QUALIFIED HYPNOTHERAPIST

When considering hypnosis for childbirth, it is essential to find a qualified and experienced hypnotherapist who specializes in working with expectant mothers. A qualified hypnotherapist should have proper certifications, training, and experience in hypnosis and specifically in the field of childbirth. They should also adhere to ethical guidelines and maintain a professional approach. To find a qualified hypnotherapist, it is recommended to seek recommendations from healthcare providers, childbirth educators, or other trusted sources. Additionally, online directories and professional associations can provide information about certified hypnotherapists in the local area. When choosing a hypnotherapist, it is important to schedule an initial consultation to discuss their approach, experience, and ensure a good fit.

Exploring hypnosis provides a deeper understanding of the nature and applications of hypnosis in the context of childbirth. Hypnosis is a natural state of focused attention that can be harnessed to promote relaxation, manage pain, and enhance the birthing experience. By dispelling common misconceptions and finding a qualified hypnotherapist, expectant mothers can confidently embrace hypnosis as a valuable tool for a positive and empowering birth journey

3.1 INTRODUCTION TO MINDFULNESS

Mindfulness is the practice of intentionally bringing one's attention to the present moment with non-judgmental awareness. It involves cultivating a state of focused attention and deepening one's connection with the present experience, including thoughts, emotions, bodily sensations, and the surrounding environment. In the context of childbirth, mindfulness can be a powerful tool for expectant mothers to navigate the various stages of pregnancy, birth, and beyond.

3.2 APPLYING MINDFULNESS IN PREGNANCY AND BIRTH

During pregnancy and birth, mindfulness can be applied in numerous ways to support expectant mothers' physical and emotional well-being. One practical application of mindfulness is through conscious breathing exercises. By focusing on the breath, expectant mothers can anchor their awareness to the present moment, fostering a sense of calm and reducing anxiety. Deep belly breathing can also promote relaxation and provide a valuable coping strategy during labor. Additionally, mindfulness can be applied to the sensations and movements of the baby in the womb. By mindfully tuning in to these experiences, mothers can cultivate a deeper connection with their unborn child and enhance the bond between them. This practice encourages expectant mothers to be fully present and appreciate the transformative journey of pregnancy.

Mindfulness also plays a significant role in preparing for birth. By being mindful of their bodies and the changes occurring during pregnancy, women can better understand their needs, seek appropriate care, and make informed decisions. Mindfulness can also help expectant mothers cultivate self-compassion, embracing the inherent wisdom of their bodies and trusting in the birthing process.

3.3 BENEFITS OF MINDFULNESS FOR EXPECTANT MOTHERS

Practicing mindfulness during pregnancy and birth offers a wide range of benefits for expectant mothers. One significant advantage is the reduction of stress and anxiety. Mindfulness helps women to approach pregnancy and birth with a sense of calm and equanimity, alleviating fears and promoting a positive mindset. By being present in the moment and focusing on their inner experiences, women can reduce the impact of stress on their physical and emotional well-being. Furthermore, mindfulness enhances self-awareness and emotional regulation. It allows expectant mothers to recognize and navigate their emotions with greater ease and resilience. By cultivating mindfulness, women can respond to the challenges of pregnancy and birth with greater clarity, adaptability, and self-compassion. Another benefit of mindfulness is the promotion of physical comfort and pain management during labor. By being fully present and adopting a non-judgmental attitude toward sensations, women can navigate the intensity of contractions and discomfort with a greater sense of acceptance and relaxation. Mindfulness-based techniques, such as body scans and mindful movement, can support women in finding positions and movements that optimize their comfort during labor.

3.4 INCORPORATING MINDFULNESS INTO DAILY LIFE

In addition to specific practices during pregnancy and birth, incorporating mindfulness into daily life can have a profound impact on the overall well-being of expectant mothers. Mindfulness is not limited to formal meditation; it can be integrated into everyday activities and moments. For example, practicing mindful eating by savoring each bite, noticing flavors, textures, and sensations, can bring a sense of nourishment and connection to the present moment. Engaging in mindful walking or gentle exercises, such as prenatal yoga, allows expectant mothers to tune in to their bodies, increase body awareness, and promote relaxation. Mindful self-care activities, such as taking warm baths, practicing self-massage, or engaging in creative expressions, can provide opportunities for nurturing and self-compassion. Moreover, establishing a regular mindfulness practice, even for a few minutes each day, can foster resilience, enhance overall well-being, and prepare expectant mothers for the demands of labor and parenthood. Mindfulness-based apps, guided meditations, and prenatal mindfulness classes can serve as valuable resources to support the incorporation of mindfulness into daily life.

Embracing mindfulness during pregnancy and birth offers expectant mothers a wealth of benefits. By cultivating present-moment awareness, managing stress, enhancing emotional well-being, and incorporating mindfulness into daily life, women can approach childbirth with greater resilience, confidence, and a deep connection to their own experiences.

4.1 DEVELOPING A POSITIVE MINDSET FOR BIRTH

Developing a positive mindset is essential for a successful Mindful Hypnobirthing experience. Expectant mothers can cultivate a positive mindset by reframing their beliefs and attitudes towards childbirth. This involves challenging any negative preconceptions or fears surrounding birth and replacing them with empowering and positive thoughts. One way to develop a positive mindset is through education and information. Learning about the physiological process of childbirth, understanding the body's capabilities, and familiarizing oneself with the stages of labor can help demystify the birthing process and instill confidence. Attending childbirth education classes or workshops specific to Mindful Hypnobirthing can provide valuable knowledge and tools to support a positive mindset.

In addition, incorporating visualization techniques can be beneficial. Creating mental images of a calm and empowered birth, visualizing the desired birth outcomes, and rehearsing positive scenarios can help shape the subconscious mind and reinforce a positive mindset. Positive affirmations, such as "I trust my body's ability to birth," can also be repeated to reinforce positive beliefs and instill confidence.

4.2 CREATING A SUPPORTIVE BIRTH PLAN

Creating a supportive birth plan is a crucial aspect of preparation for Mindful Hypnobirthing. A birth plan is a written document that outlines the expectant mother's preferences, choices, and desires regarding the birthing process. It serves as a communication tool with healthcare providers and ensures that the mother's wishes are known and respected. When creating a birth plan, it is important to include elements that align with the principles of Mindful Hypnobirthing. This may involve preferences for a calm and peaceful birthing environment, the use of specific relaxation techniques, preferences for minimal medical interventions, and promoting natural pain management strategies. Including the desire for a supportive and respectful birthing team, who are familiar with and supportive of Mindful Hypnobirthing techniques, can also be beneficial.

It is important to remember that a birth plan is a flexible guide and that unexpected circumstances may arise. Being open to changes and remaining adaptable is essential. A supportive birth partner or doula can provide valuable assistance in advocating for the mother's preferences during labor and delivery.

4.3 NURTURING A HEALTHY LIFESTYLE DURING PREGNANCY

Nurturing a healthy lifestyle during pregnancy is an integral part of Mindful Hypnobirthing preparation. A healthy lifestyle contributes to physical well-being, promotes optimal fetal development, and supports a positive birthing experience. This involves engaging in regular physical activity, consuming a balanced diet, and practicing self-care. Physical activity during pregnancy should be tailored to individual abilities and needs. Gentle exercises, such as prenatal yoga, walking, or swimming, can help maintain strength, flexibility, and promote overall well-being. It is essential to listen to one's body, modify activities as necessary, and consult with healthcare providers for guidance. Eating a balanced and nutritious diet is vital for the well-being of both the mother and the baby. This includes consuming a variety of fruits, vegetables, whole grains, lean proteins, and staying hydrated. Mindful eating practices, such as paying attention to hunger and fullness cues, savoring meals, and making conscious food choices, can enhance the connection with one's body and promote optimal nutrition.

Practicing self-care is equally important during pregnancy. This involves engaging in activities that promote relaxation, stress reduction, and emotional well-being. Mindful self-care practices, such as taking warm baths, practicing relaxation techniques, journaling, or engaging in creative outlets, can help nurture a positive mindset and support the Mindful Hypnobirthing journey.

Building a support network is crucial for expectant mothers preparing for Mindful Hypnobirthing. Surrounding oneself with a supportive community helps create a nurturing and empowering environment. This can include partners, family members, friends, or fellow expectant mothers who share similar values and are supportive of the Mindful Hypnobirthing approach.

Attending Mindful Hypnobirthing classes or workshops provides an opportunity to connect with other expectant parents who are also preparing for a calm and confident birth. These gatherings allow for the exchange of experiences, knowledge sharing, and emotional support. Online communities and social media groups dedicated to Mindful Hypnobirthing can also serve as valuable sources of support and information.

Additionally, involving the birth partner in the preparation process is essential. The birth partner can learn about Mindful Hypnobirthing techniques, practice relaxation exercises together, and provide continuous support during labor and birth. Their presence and active involvement can contribute to a positive birth experience.

Preparation for Mindful Hypnobirthing involves developing a positive mindset, creating a supportive birth plan, nurturing a healthy lifestyle, and building a strong support network. These preparations lay the foundation for a calm and confident birth experience, fostering the physical, emotional, and psychological well-being of the expectant mother.

5.1 DEEP BREATHING EXERCISES

Deep breathing exercises are a fundamental relaxation technique in Mindful Hypnobirthing. By consciously focusing on the breath, expectant mothers can tap into the body's natural relaxation response and promote a sense of calm and relaxation during pregnancy and childbirth. One deep breathing technique commonly used is diaphragmatic breathing, also known as belly breathing. This technique involves inhaling deeply through the nose, allowing the breath to expand the belly, and exhaling slowly through the mouth, allowing the belly to gently contract. This deep and intentional breathing pattern helps activate the body's relaxation response, slowing down the heart rate, reducing muscle tension, and promoting a state of calm. Another deep breathing technique is the 4-7-8 breath. It involves inhaling deeply through the nose for a count of 4, holding the breath for a count of 7, and exhaling slowly through the mouth for a count of 8. This breath pattern encourages a longer exhalation, which activates the body's relaxation response and promotes a sense of relaxation and tranquility.

Practicing deep breathing exercises regularly during pregnancy helps expectant mothers become familiar with the technique, making it easier to utilize during labor and birth. It can be beneficial to practice deep breathing in various positions, such as sitting, lying down, or during movement, to find what is most comfortable and effective for each individual.

5.2 PROGRESSIVE MUSCLE RELAXATION

Progressive Muscle Relaxation (PMR) is a relaxation technique that involves systematically tensing and releasing different muscle groups to induce a state of deep relaxation. By alternating between tensing and relaxing muscles, expectant mothers can increase body awareness, release muscle tension, and promote a sense of overall relaxation. To practice PMR, find a comfortable position and begin by tensing the muscles in one part of the body, such as the hands or feet, for a few seconds. Then, release the tension and allow the muscles to relax fully. Move on to the next muscle group, gradually working through the entire body, including the arms, shoulders, neck, face, and legs. While progressing through each muscle group, it can be helpful to focus on the sensations of tension and relaxation, cultivating a sense of mindfulness. By intentionally releasing tension and bringing awareness to each muscle group, expectant mothers can promote a deep sense of relaxation and prepare their bodies for a calm and confident birth experience.

Practicing PMR regularly during pregnancy allows expectant mothers to become familiar with the technique, making it easier to employ during labor and birth. It can also be beneficial to combine PMR with deep breathing, coordinating the release of muscle tension with the exhalation of the breath for an enhanced relaxation experience.

Guided imagery and visualizations are powerful techniques used in Mindful Hypnobirthing to create a mental landscape that promotes relaxation, confidence, and positive birth experiences. These techniques involve using the power of the mind's eye to imagine vivid and positive scenes or scenarios related to pregnancy and birth. During guided imagery exercises, expectant mothers are guided through a series of calming and empowering visualizations by either a hypnotherapist, a recorded audio, or a partner reading a script. The imagery may involve envisioning a serene natural setting, picturing oneself as a strong and capable birthing woman, or visualizing the baby's journey through the birth canal. The key to effective guided imagery and visualizations is to engage all the senses and cultivate a deep sense of immersion in the imagined scene. By incorporating details such as sounds, smells, textures, and emotions, the visualization becomes more vivid and impactful. This helps create positive neural associations and supports the body's relaxation response.

Practicing guided imagery and visualizations regularly during pregnancy enhances the effectiveness of these techniques during labor and birth. Expectant mothers can listen to pre-recorded guided imagery scripts, create their own visualizations, or seek the guidance of a trained hypnotherapist to tailor the imagery to their specific needs and preferences.

5.4 SELF-HYPNOSIS FOR RELAXATION

Self-hypnosis is a technique that allows individuals to induce a state of deep relaxation and heightened suggestibility on their own. It involves entering a trance-like state through the power of focused attention and positive suggestions. Self-hypnosis can be a valuable tool for expectant mothers to promote relaxation, manage pain, and enhance their birthing experience. To practice self-hypnosis, find a quiet and comfortable space where you can relax without interruption. Begin by using deep breathing techniques to calm the body and mind. Then, focus your attention on positive affirmations or suggestions related to relaxation, confidence, and a calm birth experience. Repeat these affirmations silently or aloud, allowing them to penetrate the subconscious mind. As you continue with self-hypnosis, you may enter a deeply relaxed state where your mind becomes highly receptive to positive suggestions. This state of heightened suggestibility allows you to harness the power of the mind-body connection, facilitating relaxation and promoting a positive mindset during pregnancy and childbirth. Regular practice of self-hypnosis during pregnancy allows expectant mothers to become more familiar with the technique and enhance their ability to enter a relaxed state at will. It is beneficial to practice self-hypnosis in various settings and positions to find what works best for each individual. Using recorded self-hypnosis audios or seeking guidance from a trained hypnotherapist can also enhance the effectiveness of self-hypnosis practice.

In conclusion, relaxation techniques play a vital role in Mindful Hypnobirthing, promoting a sense of calm, relaxation, and confidence during pregnancy and birth. Deep breathing exercises, progressive muscle relaxation, guided imagery, and self-hypnosis offer expectant mothers practical tools to support relaxation, manage discomfort, and cultivate a positive birthing experience.

Relaxation techniques play a vital role in Mindful Hypnobirthing, promoting a sense of calm, relaxation, and confidence during pregnancy and birth. Deep breathing exercises, progressive muscle relaxation, guided imagery, and self-hypnosis offer expectant mothers practical tools to support relaxation, manage discomfort, and cultivate a positive birthing experience.

6.1 USING AFFIRMATIONS FOR POSITIVE BIRTH EXPERIENCES

Affirmations are powerful statements that can help expectant mothers cultivate a positive mindset and create a sense of calm and confidence during childbirth. These positive affirmations are repeated and embraced to reprogram the subconscious mind and replace any negative beliefs or fears surrounding birth. When using affirmations, it is important to choose statements that resonate with personal beliefs and aspirations. Examples of affirmations for positive birth experiences may include "I trust my body's ability to birth," "I am relaxed and in control during labor," or "Each surge brings me closer to meeting my baby." These affirmations can be repeated silently or aloud, practiced during meditation or self-hypnosis sessions, and even written down and displayed in prominent places as constant reminders. The consistent repetition of affirmations allows the mind to accept these positive statements as true, overriding any negative thoughts or doubts. Affirmations provide expectant mothers with a source of strength and encouragement, reinforcing a belief in their own abilities and fostering a sense of empowerment throughout the birthing process.

6.2 CREATING A BIRTH VISION BOARD

A birth vision board is a visual representation of an expectant mother's desires, preferences, and aspirations for her birthing experience. It serves as a powerful tool for visualization, helping to manifest a calm and confident birth. Creating a birth vision board involves gathering images, words, and symbols that align with the desired birth experience and arranging them on a poster or a digital collage. To begin, collect magazines, printouts, or images from the internet that reflect the elements of an ideal birth experience. These can include pictures of serene natural settings, images of confident and empowered birthing women, affirmations, and symbols of strength and resilience.

Arrange these images and words on the vision board in a way that resonates with personal aesthetics and desires. Display the birth vision board in a prominent place where it can be seen daily, such as on a bedroom wall or as the screensaver on a phone or computer. Take time each day to focus on the vision board, allowing the mind to absorb the positive images and intentions. By consistently visualizing the desired birth experience through the vision board, expectant mothers create a powerful manifestation tool that reinforces their confidence and belief in a calm and confident birth.

6.3 MENTAL REHEARSAL FOR BIRTH

Mental rehearsal is a technique that involves mentally visualizing and rehearsing the entire birthing process, from early labor to the moment of meeting the baby. This practice allows expectant mothers to familiarize themselves with the sensations, emotions, and scenarios they may encounter during childbirth, and to mentally prepare for a calm and confident birth. To begin mental rehearsal, find a quiet and comfortable space where you can relax without distractions. Close your eyes and imagine the different stages of labor, envisioning the contractions, sensations, and emotions that may arise. See yourself coping with each surge in a calm and relaxed manner, utilizing relaxation techniques, breathing deeply, and trusting in your body's ability to birth. Mental rehearsal also involves envisioning the support of the birth partner, healthcare providers, and any other individuals present during the birth. Imagine their words of encouragement, their presence, and their support. Visualize a supportive and respectful birthing environment that aligns with your desires and preferences.

Practicing mental rehearsal regularly allows expectant mothers to build confidence and resilience for the birthing process. By repeatedly experiencing a calm and confident birth in the mind's eye, they create neural pathways that support a positive mindset and reinforce the belief in their ability to navigate the birthing journey.

6.4 OVERCOMING FEAR AND ANXIETY THROUGH VISUALIZATION

Visualization is a powerful technique for overcoming fear and anxiety during childbirth. By intentionally visualizing a calm and positive birth experience, expectant mothers can reframe their perception of fear, replacing it with a sense of confidence and empowerment. When experiencing fear or anxiety surrounding childbirth, take a moment to close your eyes and visualize a serene and peaceful birthing environment. Picture yourself surrounded by supportive individuals, experiencing each contraction with grace and ease. See yourself connecting with your body's natural rhythms and surrendering to the birthing process with trust and confidence. During visualization, engage all the senses to make the experience as vivid as possible. Imagine the soothing sounds, comforting scents, and gentle touch that contribute to a relaxed and calm atmosphere. Embrace the positive emotions and sensations associated with a successful and empowering birth.

Regular practice of visualization techniques allows expectant mothers to gradually release and transform fears and anxieties related to childbirth. Visualization serves as a powerful tool to reprogram the mind, enabling expectant mothers to approach birth with a sense of calm, confidence, and trust in their own abilities. Visualizing a calm and confident birth through affirmations, birth vision boards, mental rehearsal, and overcoming fear through visualization enhances the Mindful Hypnobirthing experience.

These techniques empower expectant mothers to embrace positive beliefs, foster a sense of confidence, and create an inner landscape of tranquility and empowerment as they prepare for the birth of their baby.

7.1 THE PERCEPTION OF PAIN IN CHILDBIRTH

Pain is a natural and normal part of the childbirth process. However, the perception of pain can be influenced by various factors, including fear, tension, and anxiety. It is essential to understand that pain in childbirth is subjective and unique to each individual. Some women may experience intense sensations, while others may perceive the discomfort as manageable. In Mindful Hypnobirthing, the perception of pain is approached with a focus on changing the mindset and response to pain. By promoting relaxation, reducing fear and tension, and enhancing the mind-body connection, expectant mothers can alter their perception of pain and approach it with a more positive and empowered mindset.

Hypnosis is a powerful tool for pain relief during childbirth. It allows expectant mothers to enter a deeply relaxed state where they can effectively manage sensations and discomfort. Through the power of suggestion, hypnosis can alter the perception of pain, making it more manageable and less distressing. During hypnosis, expectant mothers can employ various techniques to reduce pain sensations. This may involve visualizations, such as imagining a warm, soothing sensation flowing through the body, or using positive affirmations related to pain relief. Hypnosis can also be used to enhance the release of endorphins, the body's natural pain-relieving hormones. Working with a trained hypnotherapist or utilizing self-hypnosis techniques, expectant mothers can enter a state of deep relaxation during labor and childbirth. By accessing the subconscious mind, they can influence their perception of pain, promoting a more comfortable birthing experience.

7.3 NON-PHARMACOLOGICAL PAIN MANAGEMENT TECHNIQUES

In addition to hypnosis, Mindful Hypnobirthing offers a range of non-pharmacological pain management techniques that can be used during labor and birth. These techniques work in harmony with the body's natural processes and can enhance relaxation and pain relief. One commonly used technique is massage. Gentle massage, performed by the birth partner or a trained professional, can help relieve tension, promote relaxation, and provide a comforting touch. Massage can target specific areas of discomfort, such as the lower back or shoulders, and can be accompanied by soothing essential oils or warm compresses. Breathing techniques play a crucial role in pain management during childbirth. Deep, slow breathing and focusing on the breath can help divert attention from discomfort and promote relaxation. Techniques such as the "slow breathing technique" or "breathing through the surge" can be practiced to maintain a relaxed state during contractions.

Water immersion, commonly known as hydrotherapy, is another non-pharmacological technique that offers pain relief during labor. Immersing in warm water, such as a birthing pool or bathtub, can help alleviate discomfort, promote relaxation, and create a soothing environment. The buoyancy of water can provide relief from the pressure on the body and enhance a sense of weightlessness. Movement and position changes are valuable tools in managing pain during childbirth. Changing positions, such as walking, swaying, or adopting different birthing positions like squatting or kneeling, can help alleviate discomfort and facilitate the progress of labor.

These movements can promote optimal fetal positioning and reduce the intensity of contractions.

While non-pharmacological pain management techniques are effective for many expectant mothers, it is important to remember that pain relief options vary and should be discussed with healthcare professionals. Open communication and collaboration with the birth team can help ensure a comprehensive approach to pain management that aligns with the expectant mother's preferences and needs. Healthcare professionals can provide information about pharmacological pain relief options, such as epidurals or nitrous oxide. They can explain the benefits, risks, and potential side effects associated with these interventions. It is essential to discuss any concerns or questions with the healthcare provider to make informed decisions. In a Mindful Hypnobirthing approach, open communication with the healthcare team allows expectant mothers to explore a range of options while maintaining their desired level of control and active participation in the birthing process. It is important to remember that pain relief options can be complementary to the mindset and relaxation techniques practiced in Mindful Hypnobirthing.

Managing pain during birth is approached holistically in Mindful Hypnobirthing. By altering the perception of pain through hypnosis, utilizing non-pharmacological pain management techniques, and working collaboratively with healthcare professionals, expectant mothers can navigate the birthing process with confidence, comfort, and a sense of empowerment.

8.1 EDUCATING AND INVOLVING THE BIRTH PARTNER

The birth partner plays a vital role in supporting the expectant mother during the birthing process. In Mindful Hypnobirthing, it is crucial to educate and involve the birth partner in the preparation and practice of techniques to ensure a collaborative and supportive birthing experience. Educating the birth partner about Mindful Hypnobirthing techniques, including relaxation, breathing exercises, and visualization, helps them understand the purpose and benefits of these practices. Attending childbirth education classes together or participating in specific partner-focused Mindful Hypnobirthing workshops can provide valuable knowledge and tools to support the expectant mother during labor and birth. Involving the birth partner in regular practice sessions allows them to familiarize themselves with the techniques and actively participate in the expectant mother's preparation. This involvement creates a sense of shared responsibility and strengthens the bond between the couple, enhancing their ability to work together as a team during the birthing process.

8.2 PROVIDING EMOTIONAL SUPPORT DURING BIRTH

Emotional support is a key aspect of the birth partner's role in Mindful Hypnobirthing. During labor and birth, the birth partner can offer comfort, reassurance, and encouragement to the expectant mother, promoting a calm and positive birthing environment. Providing a nurturing and soothing presence, the birth partner can offer physical touch, such as gentle massage or holding hands, to help the expectant mother relax and manage any discomfort. Verbal affirmations and positive reinforcement can be used to remind the mother of her strength and capabilities throughout the birthing journey. Active listening is another essential skill for the birth partner. By attentively listening to the expectant mother's needs, fears, and desires, the partner can offer empathetic and supportive responses. Creating a safe and non-judgmental space for the mother to express her emotions allows her to feel understood and validated during this transformative experience.

8.3 TECHNIQUES FOR EFFECTIVE COMMUNICATION WITH THE BIRTH PARTNER

Effective communication between the expectant mother and the birth partner is vital for a harmonious and supportive birthing experience. Mindful Hypnobirthing emphasizes clear and compassionate communication to ensure that both partners feel heard, respected, and empowered. Active listening is a foundational communication technique. The birth partner can practice active listening by giving their full attention to the expectant mother, maintaining eye contact, and responding with empathy and understanding. This approach fosters a sense of trust and deepens the connection between the couple. Using positive and encouraging language is another essential aspect of effective communication. The birth partner can provide uplifting and affirming statements to reinforce the expectant mother's confidence and self-belief. Avoiding negative or fear-inducing language helps create a supportive and empowering birthing environment. Non-verbal communication is also significant during labor and birth. The birth partner can use physical touch, such as a gentle hand on the shoulder or a reassuring hug, to communicate love, support, and reassurance. Gestures and facial expressions that convey calm and confidence can help create a positive birthing atmosphere.

8.4 ENCOURAGING ACTIVE PARTICIPATION IN THE BIRTHING PROCESS

Encouraging the birth partner's active participation in the birthing process is crucial for a collaborative and empowering experience. The birth partner can actively engage in various ways to support the expectant mother during labor and birth. Assisting with relaxation techniques, such as guiding the expectant mother through breathing exercises or practicing massage techniques, allows the birth partner to actively contribute to the expectant mother's comfort and relaxation. Being present and attentive during the birthing process helps the partner understand the mother's needs and provide appropriate support. Advocacy is another essential role for the birth partner. They can communicate the expectant mother's birth preferences and wishes to healthcare professionals, ensuring that her voice is heard and respected. This advocacy includes discussing interventions, asking questions, and supporting the mother's informed decision-making. Encouraging the birth partner to trust their instincts and intuition during the birthing process is also significant. The partner can provide a source of strength and reassurance, reminding the expectant mother of her ability to birth and offering unwavering support throughout the journey.

The birth partner plays a crucial role in supporting the expectant mother during Mindful Hypnobirthing. By educating and involving the partner, providing emotional support, utilizing effective communication techniques, and encouraging active participation, the birth partner becomes an integral part of creating a calm, confident, and empowering birthing experience.

CHAPTER 9: ENHANCING BONDING AND CONNECTION

9.1 THE IMPORTANCE OF BONDING WITH YOUR BABY

Bonding with your baby is a critical aspect of the postpartum period. It fosters a deep emotional connection between the parent and the newborn, promoting the baby's sense of security, trust, and overall well-being. In Mindful Hypnobirthing, enhancing bonding and connection is emphasized as a way to nurture the parent-child relationship from the very beginning. Bonding begins immediately after birth and continues throughout the postpartum period. Spending quality time with your baby, engaging in loving and nurturing interactions, and responding to their needs helps establish a strong foundation for the parent-child bond. Mindful presence and attentive care contribute to a sense of security and attachment.

9.2 SKIN-TO-SKIN CONTACT AND ITS BENEFITS

Skin-to-skin contact, also known as kangaroo care, is a practice that involves holding your baby against your bare chest, allowing for direct skin-to-skin contact. This practice offers numerous benefits for both the parent and the newborn and is highly encouraged in Mindful Hypnobirthing.

Skin-to-skin contact immediately after birth helps regulate the baby's body temperature, stabilize their heart rate and breathing, and promote the release of bonding hormones, such as oxytocin. It creates a nurturing environment that mimics the womb, providing comfort and security for the baby. Skin-to-skin contact also facilitates the establishment of breastfeeding and supports a successful breastfeeding relationship.

Breastfeeding is not only a valuable source of nutrition for the baby but also a powerful means of enhancing bonding and connection. Mindful Hypnobirthing emphasizes promoting breastfeeding through mindful techniques that nurture the breastfeeding relationship and support the mother's confidence and well-being. Mindful breastfeeding involves being fully present and attentive during nursing sessions. It requires creating a peaceful and relaxed environment, minimizing distractions, and focusing on the intimate connection between parent and child. Mindful breathing exercises can be practiced during breastfeeding to enhance relaxation and deepen the bond. Supporting the mother's comfort during breastfeeding is essential for a positive experience. Utilizing relaxation techniques, such as deep breathing or progressive muscle relaxation, helps the mother release tension and promotes a more comfortable and enjoyable breastfeeding session. Additionally, providing emotional support, understanding, and patience fosters the mother's confidence and enhances the bonding experience.

Seeking guidance from lactation consultants or attending breastfeeding support groups can also contribute to the success of breastfeeding. These resources provide information, encouragement, and a sense of community, reinforcing the mother's commitment to breastfeeding and enhancing the connection with her baby.

In Mindful Hypnobirthing, the father's role in bonding and connection is highly valued and encouraged. Fathers can actively engage in nurturing their relationship with the baby, fostering a deep and meaningful bond from the earliest moments of the baby's life. One way to encourage father-infant bonding is through skin-to-skin contact. Fathers can also practice kangaroo care, holding the baby against their bare chest to provide a sense of comfort and security. Engaging in soothing and calming activities, such as singing, talking, or gentle massage, helps fathers establish a strong emotional connection with their newborn. Participating in caregiving activities allows fathers to bond with the baby while providing practical support to the mother. Changing diapers, bathing, or assisting with feeding create opportunities for fathers to actively engage in their child's care and deepen the parent-infant bond. Mindful presence and attentive listening are key components of father-infant bonding. By being fully present during interactions with the baby, fathers can attune to their child's cues, respond with sensitivity, and establish a strong emotional connection. Enhancing bonding and connection is essential in Mindful Hypnobirthing. Through practices such as skin-to-skin contact, promoting breastfeeding through mindful techniques, and encouraging father-infant bonding, parents can nurture a deep and loving relationship with their baby from the very beginning. These practices foster emotional well-being, support healthy development, and lay the foundation for a lifetime of connection.

Engaging in regular skin-to-skin contact beyond the immediate postpartum period continues to strengthen the bond between parent and child. It allows for intimate and comforting physical connection, promoting emotional well-being, and supporting the baby's development.

10.1 NURTURING YOUR MIND AND BODY AFTER BIRTH

The postpartum period is a time of transition and adjustment for new parents. Nurturing your mind and body during this time is essential for your well-being and the overall experience of parenthood. Mindful Hypnobirthing emphasizes the importance of self-care practices that support postpartum recovery. Rest and sleep are crucial aspects of postpartum recovery. Prioritize getting enough rest and create a sleep-friendly environment. Nap when the baby sleeps and ask for support from your partner or loved ones to ensure you have adequate time to recharge. Nutrition plays a vital role in postpartum healing. Focus on nourishing your body with nutrient-dense foods that support recovery and breastfeeding if applicable. Stay hydrated and include foods rich in vitamins, minerals, and healthy fats to promote physical and emotional well-being.

10.2 MINDFUL PRACTICES FOR POSTPARTUM HEALING

Mindful practices can help facilitate postpartum healing and support emotional well-being during this transitional period. Incorporate mindfulness techniques into your daily routine to promote self-care and enhance your overall postpartum experience. Mindful breathing exercises can provide moments of calm and relaxation amidst the demands of parenthood. Take a few deep breaths, focusing on the sensations of the breath as it enters and leaves your body. This practice can help alleviate stress, promote a sense of grounding, and enhance overall well-being. Practicing self-compassion is essential during the postpartum period. Embrace the imperfections and challenges that come with parenthood and offer yourself kindness and understanding. Be patient with your own healing process, both physically and emotionally, and allow yourself to ask for help when needed.

Journaling can be a valuable tool for self-reflection and emotional processing. Take a few minutes each day to write down your thoughts, emotions, and experiences. This practice provides an outlet for self-expression and can help cultivate self-awareness and a deeper understanding of your postpartum journey.

10.3 BALANCING SELF-CARE WITH THE DEMANDS OF PARENTHOOD

Balancing self-care with the demands of parenthood can be challenging, but it is crucial for your well-being and the ability to care for your baby. Mindful Hypnobirthing encourages finding a balance that nourishes both your needs and those of your child. Set realistic expectations and avoid putting pressure on yourself to do everything perfectly. Prioritize self-care activities that replenish your energy and promote your overall well-being. This might include taking short breaks for self-reflection or engaging in activities that bring you joy and relaxation. Delegate tasks and accept support from your partner, family members, or friends. Communicate your needs and ask for help when necessary. Recognize that it takes a village to raise a child, and accepting assistance allows you to focus on your own recovery and self-care.

10.4 SEEKING SUPPORT DURING THE POSTPARTUM PERIOD

Seeking support is crucial during the postpartum period. Connect with other parents who are going through similar experiences, either through support groups or online communities. Sharing your thoughts and feelings can provide validation and a sense of camaraderie. Consider reaching out to healthcare professionals, such as lactation consultants or postpartum doulas, who can offer guidance and support specific to your needs. These professionals can address any concerns or challenges you may be facing and provide resources to support your postpartum recovery and adjustment to parenthood. Remember that seeking support is not a sign of weakness but a reflection of your commitment to your own well-being and the well-being of your family.

In conclusion, postpartum recovery and self-care are essential components of the Mindful Hypnobirthing journey. Nurturing your mind and body, incorporating mindful practices, balancing self-care with the demands of parenthood, and seeking support contribute to a positive and fulfilling postpartum experience. By prioritizing your well-being, you can navigate the challenges and joys of early parenthood with greater ease and resilience.

11.1 APPLYING MINDFULNESS IN PARENTING

Mindful parenting involves bringing the principles of mindfulness to the relationship between parent and child. It is about being fully present, non-judgmental, and accepting of both yourself and your child. Applying mindfulness in parenting allows for greater connection, empathy, and understanding. To practice mindful parenting, bring your attention to the present moment when interacting with your child. Engage in activities together without distractions, such as putting away electronic devices and giving your child your undivided attention. By being fully present, you can observe and appreciate your child's unique qualities and experiences. Acceptance is a core aspect of mindful parenting. Recognize and embrace your child for who they are, without trying to change or control them. This acceptance fosters a sense of safety and unconditional love, creating a strong foundation for their emotional well-being and development.

11.2 MINDFUL COMMUNICATION WITH YOUR CHILD

Mindful communication with your child involves listening and speaking with awareness and compassion. It is about being attuned to your child's needs and emotions, while also expressing yourself in a way that promotes understanding and connection. Active listening is an essential component of mindful communication. Be fully present and attentive when your child is speaking to you. Offer them your undivided attention, maintain eye contact, and listen without judgment or interruption. Reflect back on what they say to ensure understanding and to validate their feelings. When expressing yourself to your child, use clear and compassionate language. Be mindful of the tone and volume of your voice, as well as your body language. Communicate with respect and empathy, considering your child's age and developmental stage. Mindful communication promotes healthy parent-child relationships and helps build trust and emotional closeness.

11.3 SUPPORTING YOUR CHILD'S EMOTIONAL WELL-BEING

Supporting your child's emotional well-being is a vital aspect of mindful parenting. It involves creating a nurturing and emotionally safe environment where your child feels comfortable expressing their feelings and experiences. Validate your child's emotions by acknowledging and accepting their feelings, even if you may not fully understand or agree with them. Encourage open communication and provide a listening ear when they want to share their thoughts and concerns. By doing so, you help your child develop emotional intelligence and resilience. Teach your child mindfulness techniques that can support their emotional well-being. For example, guide them in deep breathing exercises or introduce simple mindfulness activities tailored to their age, such as mindful coloring or body scans. These practices help your child cultivate self-awareness, emotional regulation, and a sense of inner calm.

11.4 INCORPORATING MINDFULNESS INTO FAMILY LIFE

Incorporating mindfulness into family life creates a harmonious and connected environment. It involves finding opportunities to practice mindfulness together as a family and to foster a sense of shared presence and well-being. Create moments of mindfulness in daily routines, such as mealtimes or bedtime rituals. Encourage the family to eat together mindfully, savoring each bite and engaging in conversation. Before bedtime, practice a short guided meditation or engage in a calming activity to promote relaxation and quality sleep. Engage in mindful activities as a family, such as going for nature walks, practicing yoga together, or participating in mindful crafts. These activities encourage connection, creativity, and shared moments of presence. Set healthy boundaries around technology use within the family. Establish designated times and spaces for device-free activities, allowing everyone to unplug and fully engage with one another.

This practice fosters meaningful connections and reduces distractions. By incorporating mindfulness into family life, you create an environment that supports emotional well-being, positive communication, and deep connections between family members.

Mindful parenting and child development go hand in hand. By applying mindfulness in parenting, practicing mindful communication, supporting your child's emotional well-being, and incorporating mindfulness into family life, you nurture a loving, compassionate, and connected family dynamic. These practices promote healthy child development and contribute to the well-being of the entire family.

12.1 COPING WITH UNEXPECTED CHANGES DURING BIRTH

Childbirth is a dynamic process, and unexpected changes can arise. Coping with these changes mindfully can help navigate challenging situations and maintain a positive mindset. One essential aspect of coping with unexpected changes is to stay informed and educated about various birth scenarios. Attend childbirth education classes or seek out resources that provide information about different interventions and procedures. Understanding the potential changes that may occur during birth can alleviate fear and anxiety and empower you to make informed decisions. Practicing flexibility and adapting to changing circumstances is crucial. Remember that birth is a unique journey, and being open to adjustments can lead to positive outcomes. Utilize the mindfulness techniques you have learned to stay present, calm, and focused on your well-being and the well-being of your baby. Seek support from your birth team, including your healthcare provider, doula, or birthing partner. Communicate your concerns and desires, and work together to create a plan that aligns with your values and preferences. Having a supportive and knowledgeable team can provide guidance and reassurance during unexpected changes.

12.2 MANAGING INDUCTIONS AND MEDICAL INTERVENTIONS MINDFULLY

Inductions and medical interventions may become necessary during childbirth. Managing these interventions mindfully can help you feel empowered and maintain a sense of control over your birth experience. If an induction is recommended, take time to understand the reasons and potential benefits and risks. Discuss the process with your healthcare provider and ask questions to clarify any concerns. Engage in relaxation techniques, such as deep breathing or visualization, to promote a calm state of mind during the induction process. During medical interventions, stay present and focused on your body and baby. Utilize mindfulness techniques to manage any discomfort or anxiety that may arise. Practice deep breathing and positive affirmations to promote relaxation and a positive mindset. Maintain open communication with your birth team. Express your preferences and concerns, and work together to ensure that your voice is heard and respected. Creating a collaborative relationship with your healthcare provider fosters a sense of trust and empowerment during medical interventions.

12.3 DEALING WITH UNPLANNED CESAREAN BIRTHS

In some cases, a cesarean birth may become necessary, even if it was not initially part of your birth plan. Coping with an unplanned cesarean birth mindfully can help you navigate the emotional and physical aspects of the experience. Acknowledge your feelings and allow yourself to process any disappointment or sadness that may arise. Remember that your primary goal is the health and well-being of yourself and your baby. Practice self-compassion and embrace the reality of the situation with understanding and acceptance. Discuss the reasons for the cesarean birth with your healthcare provider to gain clarity and understanding. Engage in open communication and ask any questions you may have. Seek support from your birth partner, family, or friends to process your emotions and provide you with comfort. Utilize mindfulness techniques to support your healing and recovery. Focus on deep breathing, gentle movements, and visualization to promote relaxation and aid in physical and emotional healing. Connect with your baby through skin-to-skin contact and breastfeeding, fostering a sense of bonding and connection.

Join support groups or seek out resources specifically tailored to cesarean birth recovery. Connecting with others who have had similar experiences can provide validation, support, and guidance throughout your healing journey.

Postpartum mental health is a significant concern for many new parents. Mindful healing during the postpartum period involves prioritizing your mental well-being, seeking support, and engaging in self-care practices. Monitor your emotional well-being and be aware of any signs of postpartum depression, anxiety, or other mental health conditions. Reach out to healthcare professionals who can provide guidance and support. Remember that seeking help is a sign of strength and is essential for your well-being and the well-being of your family. Incorporate self-care practices into your daily routine. This may include engaging in activities that bring you joy and relaxation, prioritizing rest and sleep, nourishing your body with healthy foods, and participating in gentle exercises that support your physical and mental well-being. Practice self-compassion and let go of any expectations of perfection. Embrace the challenges and joys of parenthood with understanding and acceptance. Cultivate a supportive network of family and friends who can provide emotional support and practical assistance when needed. Engage in mindfulness and meditation practices to support your mental health. Set aside time each day to focus on your breath, bring awareness to the present moment, and cultivate a sense of calm and peace. Mindful parenting and self-compassion practices can also contribute to your overall well-being.

Addressing common concerns and challenges mindfully allows for greater resilience, acceptance, and empowerment during childbirth and the postpartum period. By approaching unexpected changes, managing medical interventions, navigating unplanned cesarean births, and prioritizing postpartum mental health, you can cultivate a positive and mindful healing journey.

13.1 MINDFUL TECHNIQUES FOR HIGH-RISK PREGNANCIES

High-risk pregnancies present unique challenges, and practicing Mindful Hypnobirthing can provide valuable support during this time. It is important to work closely with your healthcare provider to develop a comprehensive plan that addresses your specific needs and ensures the safety and well-being of both you and your baby. Mindful techniques can help manage stress and anxiety that may arise during a high-risk pregnancy. Deep breathing exercises, meditation, and visualization can promote relaxation and a sense of calm. These techniques can be practiced regularly to cultivate a positive mindset and help you navigate the uncertainties that come with a high-risk pregnancy. Engage in open and honest communication with your healthcare provider. Discuss your fears, concerns, and desires for your birth experience. Collaborate with your healthcare team to create a plan that addresses any potential complications and ensures that you are well-informed and supported throughout the process. Utilize affirmations and positive self-talk to reinforce your confidence and resilience. Affirmations can be tailored to your specific circumstances, focusing on affirming the strength and health of yourself and your baby. Repeat these affirmations regularly, allowing them to become a source of empowerment and encouragement. Seek out additional support through support groups or online communities.

Connecting with others who have experienced or are currently going through a high-risk pregnancy can provide validation, understanding, and valuable insights. Sharing your journey with others who can relate to your experiences can help alleviate feelings of isolation and provide a sense of camaraderie.

13.2 HYPNOSIS AND MINDFULNESS FOR TWIN OR MULTIPLE BIRTHS

Twin or multiple births bring their own set of considerations, and Mindful Hypnobirthing can be adapted to support expectant parents in these special circumstances. Hypnosis and mindfulness techniques can help promote relaxation, manage anxiety, and support a positive birth experience. Deep relaxation techniques, such as guided imagery and progressive muscle relaxation, can be especially beneficial for managing the physical and emotional demands of carrying multiple babies. Regularly engaging in these practices can help you find a sense of calm and balance as you prepare for the birth of your twins or multiples. Develop a comprehensive birth plan with the guidance of your healthcare provider. Discuss options for birthing positions, pain management, and interventions specific to twin or multiple births. By understanding the unique considerations of multiple pregnancies, you can make informed decisions that align with your birth preferences. Practice mindful bonding with each of your babies throughout your pregnancy. Take time to connect with each individual baby, nurturing a sense of love and connection. Engage in activities that promote bonding, such as talking, singing, or gentle touch, while keeping in mind the comfort and safety of both you and your babies.

Utilize visualizations that encompass the birth of your twins or multiples. Envision a calm and supportive birthing environment, with each baby progressing safely and smoothly. Visualize yourself feeling confident, empowered, and supported as you bring your babies into the world.

13.3 SUPPORTING BIRTH AFTER TRAUMATIC EXPERIENCES

For those who have experienced traumatic births in the past, Mindful Hypnobirthing can offer support and healing during subsequent pregnancies. It is important to address any unresolved emotions or fears surrounding the previous traumatic experience to promote a positive and empowering birth journey. Seek professional support, such as therapy or counseling, to process and heal from previous birth trauma. A trained therapist can guide you through trauma-focused therapy techniques, helping you navigate any unresolved emotions and fears related to your past experience. Engage in self-care practices that prioritize your emotional well-being. This may include activities such as journaling, meditation, or engaging in creative outlets that promote self-expression. Mindful self-compassion practices can also help you cultivate a positive and nurturing mindset as you prepare for your upcoming birth. Develop a birth plan that reflects your preferences and addresses your specific concerns. Collaborate with your healthcare provider and any other members of your birth team to create a supportive and empowering environment. Open communication is essential in ensuring that your needs and desires are understood and respected throughout the birthing process. Consider utilizing hypnosis as a tool for relaxation and healing. Hypnosis can help release fear and tension associated with past trauma and promote a positive mindset. Working with a trained hypnotherapist experienced in supporting individuals with birth trauma can be particularly beneficial.

13.4 MINDFUL HYPNOBIRTHING FOR VBAC (VAGINAL BIRTH AFTER CESAREAN)

Vaginal Birth after Cesarean (VBAC) can be a unique and empowering choice for expectant parents. Mindful Hypnobirthing techniques can provide support and confidence as you navigate the journey towards a successful VBAC. Educate yourself about the specific considerations and risks associated with VBAC. Discuss your desire for a VBAC with your healthcare provider, ensuring that you meet the necessary criteria and that your healthcare team is supportive of your decision. Engage in mindful relaxation techniques to manage any fears or anxieties related to your VBAC. Practice deep breathing, guided imagery, and positive affirmations to cultivate a sense of calm and confidence. Visualize a smooth and successful VBAC, focusing on your body's ability to birth your baby naturally. Utilize the power of self-hypnosis to release any lingering fear or tension surrounding your previous cesarean birth. By working with a trained hypnotherapist or utilizing self-hypnosis techniques, you can reframe your mindset and approach the VBAC experience with a positive and empowered attitude. Assemble a supportive birth team that is experienced in supporting VBACs. Collaborate with your healthcare provider, doula, or midwife to create a birth plan that aligns with your preferences and maximizes your chances of a successful VBAC. Their expertise and encouragement can provide reassurance and guidance throughout the process. Mindful Hypnobirthing can be adapted to various special circumstances, offering support and empowerment in high-risk pregnancies, twin or multiple births, birth after trauma, and VBAC journeys. By incorporating mindfulness techniques, utilizing hypnosis, seeking support, and working closely with your healthcare team, you can navigate these unique circumstances with confidence and mindfulness.

14.1 FINDING MINDFUL HYPNOBIRTHING CLASSES OR WORKSHOPS

Attending Mindful Hypnobirthing classes or workshops can be a valuable way to deepen your understanding, practice techniques, and connect with like-minded individuals. Finding local classes or workshops can be done through various channels. Start by asking your healthcare provider, midwife, or doula for recommendations. They may be familiar with practitioners or organizations that offer Mindful Hypnobirthing classes in your area. Hospitals, birthing centers, and holistic health centers may also offer courses or have information on upcoming workshops. Online research can also help you find Mindful Hypnobirthing classes near you. Search for keywords such as "Mindful Hypnobirthing classes" or "Hypnobirthing workshops" along with your location. This can lead you to local practitioners or organizations that offer in-person instruction. Consider attending introductory sessions or free informational events to get a sense of the teaching style and approach of different practitioners. This can help you determine which instructor resonates with you and aligns with your values and goals for your birth experience. Additionally, some Mindful Hypnobirthing instructors offer online classes or workshops, which can provide flexibility and accessibility, especially if local options are limited. Online platforms and directories dedicated to childbirth education may have listings for virtual Mindful Hypnobirthing classes that you can participate in from the comfort of your own home.

Online communities and support groups can be invaluable resources for connecting with others on the Mindful Hypnobirthing journey. These platforms provide spaces to share experiences, seek advice, and offer support to fellow parents-to-be. Social media platforms like Facebook, Instagram, and Twitter often have dedicated groups or hashtags related to Mindful Hypnobirthing. Joining these groups allows you to engage in conversations, ask questions, and receive support from a community of like-minded individuals. You can share your own experiences, gain insights from others, and find encouragement throughout your preparation and birthing process. Online forums and discussion boards centered around childbirth and Mindful Hypnobirthing can also provide a wealth of information and support. Platforms such as BabyCenter, Reddit, or specialized childbirth forums often have dedicated threads or sections for discussing Mindful Hypnobirthing. Engaging in these forums can help you connect with individuals who have similar interests and concerns. When participating in online communities, remember that everyone's experiences are unique. Seek evidence-based information and advice, and always consult with your healthcare provider for personalized guidance. Respect the diversity of opinions and experiences within the community, and maintain a supportive and compassionate approach to discussions.

14.3 CONNECTING WITH OTHER MINDFUL HYPNOBIRTHING PARENTS

Connecting with other Mindful Hypnobirthing parents can be a powerful way to share experiences, gain insights, and build a support network. Forming connections with individuals who have gone through or are going through a similar journey can provide validation, inspiration, and encouragement. Consider attending local or virtual meetups, workshops, or events specifically focused on Mindful Hypnobirthing. These gatherings provide opportunities to connect with other parents and engage in meaningful conversations about childbirth, parenting, and mindfulness. Additionally, online platforms and social media groups mentioned earlier can be effective tools for finding and connecting with other Mindful Hypnobirthing parents. Engage in conversations, ask questions, and share your own experiences. Building relationships with others who understand and support your approach to childbirth can be empowering and uplifting. Mindful Hypnobirthing practitioners may also organize group sessions or support circles for their clients. Inquire with your instructor about any community-building activities they offer. These sessions provide a space for sharing, learning, and connecting with others who are on a similar path.

Remember that every birth experience is unique, and connecting with others does not mean that your journey will be identical to theirs. Embrace the diversity of experiences and perspectives within the Mindful Hypnobirthing community, and approach connections with curiosity, empathy, and respect.

In conclusion, there are various resources and support networks available to enhance your Mindful Hypnobirthing journey. Books, websites, apps, classes, online communities, and connections with other parents can provide valuable information, guidance, and a sense of community. Utilize these resources to deepen your understanding, gain support, and build confidence as you prepare for your calm and confident birth.

15.1 STORIES OF EMPOWERED AND POSITIVE BIRTHS

Real-life experiences of Mindful Hypnobirthing can inspire and encourage expectant parents on their own birthing journeys. Hearing stories of empowered and positive births can instill confidence and demonstrate the potential of Mindful Hypnobirthing techniques in creating a calm and positive birthing experience. One such story is that of Sarah, who practiced Mindful Hypnobirthing throughout her pregnancy and birth. Sarah diligently practiced deep breathing, relaxation techniques, and affirmations. During her labor, she remained calm and focused, allowing her body to work naturally. With the support of her partner and birth team, Sarah gave birth to her baby boy in a peaceful and empowered manner. Sarah attributes her positive birth experience to the mindfulness and hypnosis techniques she learned, which helped her trust her body and surrender to the birthing process. Another empowering birth story is that of Michael and Emily, who chose Mindful Hypnobirthing for their home birth. They created a tranquil birthing environment, utilizing soothing music, dim lighting, and aromatherapy. Through mindfulness and hypnosis techniques, Emily was able to relax deeply and work with her body's natural rhythms. Michael provided unwavering support, utilizing massage and encouraging affirmations. Together, they welcomed their baby girl into the world with a deep sense of joy and connection.

These stories demonstrate the potential of Mindful Hypnobirthing in fostering positive, empowering birth experiences. They highlight the importance of preparation, practice, and support in creating an environment conducive to calm and confident birthing.

15.2 OVERCOMING CHALLENGES THROUGH MINDFUL HYPNOBIRTHING

Mindful Hypnobirthing can provide valuable tools for overcoming challenges that may arise during labor and birth. These techniques can help individuals maintain a sense of control, cope with unexpected situations, and navigate potential obstacles. Consider the story of Emma, who experienced a longer labor than anticipated. Despite fatigue and moments of doubt, Emma relied on her Mindful Hypnobirthing practices to stay calm and focused. She practiced deep relaxation, visualization, and affirmations, which helped her manage the intensity of contractions and maintain a positive mindset. With the support of her birth team and her own determination, Emma ultimately birthed her baby boy with a deep sense of accomplishment and resilience. Another example is that of Mark and Sarah, who faced a change in birth plans due to medical reasons. They had prepared for a home birth but needed to transfer to the hospital during labor. Through their Mindful Hypnobirthing practice, they remained centered and adaptable. They continued to utilize relaxation techniques, affirmations, and mindful breathing in the hospital setting, creating a calm and serene atmosphere despite the change in surroundings. This allowed them to navigate the unexpected with grace and confidence, ultimately birthing their baby girl in a positive and supported environment.

These case studies demonstrate how Mindful Hypnobirthing can help individuals adapt to unexpected challenges and maintain a positive mindset during labor and birth. The tools and techniques learned through Mindful Hypnobirthing can provide a sense of empowerment and resilience, enabling individuals to navigate any twists and turns that may arise during the birthing process.

Every birth journey is unique, and each experience offers valuable lessons and insights. By examining a variety of birth journeys, we can gain a deeper understanding of the range of possibilities and the ways in which Mindful Hypnobirthing can positively impact different circumstances. One important lesson learned is the significance of preparation. Practicing Mindful Hypnobirthing techniques throughout pregnancy helps individuals build confidence, deepen their understanding of the birthing process, and establish a strong foundation for a positive birth experience. Through consistent practice, individuals become familiar with relaxation techniques, affirmations, and visualization, allowing them to integrate these tools effortlessly during labor and birth. Another lesson is the power of support and connection. Having a supportive birth team, including partners, doulas, or healthcare providers, plays a crucial role in maintaining a positive birthing environment. The presence of a knowledgeable and understanding support system can provide encouragement, guidance, and reassurance throughout the birthing journey. Flexibility and adaptability are also important lessons to embrace. Birth plans may need to be adjusted, unexpected situations may arise, and individuals must be prepared to go with the flow. Mindful Hypnobirthing equips individuals with the ability to remain present, adaptable, and open to whatever unfolds during labor and birth. Lastly, the significance of self-belief and trust in the birthing process cannot be overstated. By cultivating a positive mindset and embracing the innate wisdom of the body, individuals can tap into their inner strength and birth their babies with confidence and grace. Trusting in the body's ability to birth and surrendering to the birthing process can profoundly impact the overall birthing experience. These lessons highlight the transformative potential of Mindful Hypnobirthing in various birth journeys. By being open to the lessons learned from others' experiences, expectant parents can gain valuable insights that empower them on their own unique birthing paths.

15.4 INSPIRING TESTIMONIALS FROM MINDFUL HYPNOBIRTHING PRACTITIONERS

Testimonials from Mindful Hypnobirthing practitioners provide firsthand accounts of the transformative power of this approach to childbirth. These stories illustrate the profound impact that Mindful Hypnobirthing can have on the birthing experiences of both practitioners and their clients. Emma, a certified Mindful Hypnobirthing practitioner, shares her own personal journey of using these techniques during the birth of her daughter. She recounts how practicing mindfulness and self-hypnosis allowed her to remain calm and relaxed throughout labor. By surrendering to the birthing process and trusting her body, she experienced a birth that was both empowering and beautiful. Inspired by her own experience, Emma became a practitioner to help other parents discover the potential of Mindful

Hypnobirthing for their own birth journeys. Sarah, another practitioner, describes her work with clients and the positive impact that Mindful Hypnobirthing has had on their births. She recounts stories of clients who were able to manage their pain effectively, maintain a deep sense of calm, and birth their babies with confidence and joy. Sarah emphasizes the importance of practice and preparation, noting that consistent use of Mindful Hypnobirthing techniques helps individuals cultivate the skills and mindset necessary for a positive birth experience. Alex, a father who attended Mindful Hypnobirthing classes with his partner, shares his perspective on the impact of these practices. He recalls how learning mindfulness and relaxation techniques enabled him to provide effective support during labor. By practicing mindful communication and offering words of affirmation, he was able to create a calm and encouraging environment for his partner. Alex emphasizes the transformative effect that Mindful Hypnobirthing had on his own confidence and connection with his partner throughout the birthing process. These testimonials highlight the personal experiences and insights of Mindful Hypnobirthing practitioners and those who have experienced its benefits. They showcase the empowerment, confidence, and deep connection that can be cultivated through Mindful Hypnobirthing practices. The testimonials also reflect the diversity of birth experiences and circumstances in which Mindful Hypnobirthing has proven effective. Whether it is a natural birth, a birth involving medical interventions, a high-risk pregnancy, or a VBAC, the principles and techniques of Mindful Hypnobirthing have been shown to positively influence the birth experience. By sharing these inspiring testimonials, expectant parents can gain a deeper understanding of the possibilities and potential benefits of Mindful Hypnobirthing. These firsthand accounts offer reassurance, inspiration, and a sense of community for those considering or embarking on their own Mindful Hypnobirthing journey. The testimonials from Mindful Hypnobirthing practitioners provide personal and inspiring accounts of the transformative power of this approach to childbirth. These stories highlight the profound impact that Mindful Hypnobirthing can have on individuals, couples, and families as they navigate the birthing process with confidence, calm, and joy.

CHAPTER 16: INTEGRATING MINDFUL HYPNOBIRTHING INTO TRADITIONAL BIRTH SETTINGS

16.1 COLLABORATING WITH HEALTHCARE PROVIDERS

Integrating Mindful Hypnobirthing into traditional birth settings involves collaboration between expectant parents, Mindful Hypnobirthing practitioners, and healthcare providers. Open and respectful communication is key to ensuring that all parties involved are aligned in their approach to creating a positive and supportive birth environment.

Start by initiating conversations with your healthcare provider about your interest in practicing Mindful Hypnobirthing during your birth. Share your goals, desires, and the techniques you plan to use. Discuss how Mindful Hypnobirthing can complement existing medical practices and interventions. Collaboratively explore ways to integrate Mindful Hypnobirthing techniques into your birth plan, while still prioritizing the safety and well-being of both you and your baby. It can be beneficial to provide educational resources on Mindful Hypnobirthing to your healthcare provider. This can include books, articles, or reputable websites that explain the principles and techniques of Mindful Hypnobirthing. By sharing evidence-based information, you can help bridge any knowledge gaps and facilitate a deeper understanding of the benefits and practices associated with Mindful Hypnobirthing. Encourage open dialogue between your Mindful Hypnobirthing practitioner and your healthcare provider. This allows for a comprehensive understanding of your birthing preferences and the integration of Mindful Hypnobirthing techniques into the care you receive. A collaborative approach ensures that everyone involved is working together to create a supportive and positive birth experience.

Educating maternity staff about Mindful Hypnobirthing is essential for creating a cohesive and supportive birth environment. By sharing knowledge and insights with the healthcare professionals who will be involved in your birth, you can enhance their understanding of Mindful Hypnobirthing and its role in promoting a calm and positive birth experience. Consider providing educational materials, such as pamphlets or handouts, that explain the basic principles and techniques of Mindful Hypnobirthing. These materials can be distributed to maternity staff, including nurses, midwives, and obstetricians, to facilitate a better understanding of how Mindful Hypnobirthing can enhance the birthing process. Arrange for a meeting or presentation with the maternity staff to discuss Mindful Hypnobirthing in more detail. Invite your Mindful Hypnobirthing practitioner to speak about the techniques, benefits, and experiences associated with this approach. This presentation can include demonstrations of relaxation techniques and provide an opportunity for staff to ask questions and engage in meaningful discussions. Encourage healthcare providers to attend Mindful Hypnobirthing workshops or training sessions to gain a firsthand experience of the techniques and their potential benefits. This can help foster a deeper appreciation and integration of Mindful Hypnobirthing into their approach to maternity care.

Continual communication and feedback with the maternity staff are crucial. Encourage dialogue about how Mindful Hypnobirthing can be integrated into routine care practices and interventions. By maintaining an open and collaborative relationship with the maternity staff, you can ensure that the birthing environment remains supportive and aligned with your Mindful Hypnobirthing goals.

16.3 ADAPTING MINDFUL TECHNIQUES IN HOSPITAL OR BIRTHING CENTER ENVIRONMENTS

Integrating Mindful Hypnobirthing techniques into hospital or birthing center environments may require some adaptation. While these settings may have different protocols and procedures, it is possible to create a calming and supportive atmosphere that aligns with the principles of Mindful Hypnobirthing. Create a birth environment that promotes relaxation and calmness. Dim the lights, play soothing music, and utilize aromatherapy, if permitted. These elements can help create a tranquil atmosphere and facilitate a sense of relaxation and focus. Discuss the use of movement and positioning during labor with your healthcare provider. Many hospitals and birthing centers are supportive of various birthing positions that promote comfort and optimal fetal positioning. Practice and incorporate positions that are conducive to relaxation, such as kneeling, sitting on a birth ball, or using a birthing stool.

Utilize visualization and guided imagery during medical procedures or interventions. For example, if an epidural is necessary, imagine the anesthesia flowing smoothly and bringing comfort to your body. By incorporating visualization techniques, you can create a positive narrative around medical interventions, helping to reduce fear and anxiety. Collaborate with your healthcare provider to explore options for a calm and gentle cesarean birth, if needed. Discuss the possibility of a "gentle cesarean" where elements such as a clear drape, immediate skin-to-skin contact, and a calm birthing atmosphere are prioritized. These adaptations can help create a more mindful and empowering cesarean birth experience.

Work with your healthcare provider to incorporate uninterrupted skin-to-skin contact and early breastfeeding initiation. These practices support bonding, regulate newborn temperature, and facilitate the establishment of breastfeeding.

Creating a supportive birth atmosphere in traditional birth settings involves collaboration with healthcare providers, birth partners, and the birthing team. By fostering a positive and compassionate atmosphere, expectant parents can enhance their Mindful Hypnobirthing experience and create a supportive environment for their birthing journey. Communicate your birth preferences clearly and assertively. Share your desires for a calm and positive birth experience with your healthcare provider and birth team. Discuss the importance of minimal interruptions, limited conversation, and a peaceful environment during labor. Designate a birth partner or support person to advocate for your preferences during labor. This individual can help maintain the birthing atmosphere, communicate your needs to the birthing team, and provide continuous support and encouragement. Consider creating a birth playlist of calming music that resonates with you and promotes relaxation. Discuss with your healthcare provider and birthing team the option of playing this music during labor to create a soothing and peaceful ambiance. Encourage the use of gentle touch and massage during labor. Discuss with your birth partner or support person techniques that provide comfort and relaxation. This physical support can help release tension and promote a deeper state of relaxation. Utilize affirmations and visualizations throughout labor to maintain a positive mindset. Write down affirmations that resonate with you and read them aloud or have your birth partner recite them to you during contractions. Visualize your baby's descent and birth, imagining a calm and gentle journey. Request minimal medical interventions, if appropriate for your situation. Share your desire for a natural and unmedicated birth experience, while remaining open to the guidance and expertise of your healthcare provider. By collaborating with healthcare providers, educating maternity staff, adapting techniques to the birth setting, and creating a supportive birth atmosphere, expectant parents can successfully integrate Mindful Hypnobirthing into traditional birth settings. This collaborative approach allows for a cohesive and respectful birthing environment that supports a calm and positive birth experience.

17.1 TRAINING AND CERTIFICATION IN MINDFUL HYPNOBIRTHING

For birth professionals, obtaining training and certification in Mindful Hypnobirthing can be a valuable addition to their skill set. Training programs and certification courses provide birth professionals with the knowledge and tools necessary to support expectant parents who choose to incorporate Mindful Hypnobirthing into their birth experiences. Look for reputable training programs that offer comprehensive instruction in Mindful Hypnobirthing techniques. These programs typically cover topics such as relaxation techniques, self-hypnosis, visualization, affirmations, and the principles of mindfulness in childbirth. Training programs may also include modules on the science behind Mindful Hypnobirthing, birth physiology, and the integration of Mindful Hypnobirthing into traditional birth settings.

Upon completing a training program, birth professionals can pursue certification in Mindful Hypnobirthing. Certification serves as a testament to their expertise and dedication to supporting individuals and couples through the Mindful Hypnobirthing approach. Certification also provides credibility and reassurance to clients seeking practitioners knowledgeable in Mindful Hypnobirthing techniques. Continuing education and professional development are essential for birth professionals working with Mindful Hypnobirthing. Attend workshops, conferences, and webinars that focus on the latest research, techniques, and best practices in Mindful Hypnobirthing. By staying updated with current information and ongoing learning, birth professionals can provide the best possible support to their clients.

Doula practices naturally align with the principles of Mindful Hypnobirthing, making it a valuable addition to the services offered by doulas. Doulas who incorporate Mindful Hypnobirthing techniques into their practice can provide holistic support to expectant parents before, during, and after birth. As a doula, seek out Mindful Hypnobirthing training and certification to gain a deep understanding of the techniques and principles involved. This knowledge will enhance your ability to guide and support clients who choose to practice Mindful Hypnobirthing during their birth experiences. Work closely with expectant parents to develop birth plans that incorporate Mindful Hypnobirthing techniques. Discuss their preferences, desires, and goals for their birth, and offer guidance on how Mindful Hypnobirthing can be integrated into their specific circumstances. During labor, provide continuous support to clients using Mindful Hypnobirthing techniques. Utilize relaxation techniques, affirmations, and visualizations to help clients maintain a calm and focused mindset. Offer gentle reminders and cues to help them stay connected to their practice during the intensity of labor. Collaborate with healthcare providers and the birthing team to ensure that the birth environment supports the Mindful Hypnobirthing approach. Advocate for your client's preferences and create a peaceful and supportive atmosphere that aligns with their Mindful Hypnobirthing goals.

Support clients in utilizing Mindful Hypnobirthing techniques to cope with challenges or changes in their birth plans. Help them adapt their practice, provide reassurance, and offer emotional support during any unexpected circumstances.

As a birth professional, supporting clients through Mindful Hypnobirthing techniques involves empowering them to cultivate a positive and confident mindset, facilitating their practice of relaxation and visualization, and providing ongoing emotional support throughout their birth journey. Empower clients by educating them about the benefits and principles of Mindful Hypnobirthing. Explain the mind-body connection, the role of relaxation in pain management, and the power of positive affirmations. Help them understand the physiological processes of labor and birth, empowering them with knowledge to make informed decisions. Guide clients in developing personalized affirmations and visualizations that resonate with them. Encourage them to practice these techniques regularly during pregnancy to establish familiarity and comfort. Offer suggestions and examples based on their unique circumstances and preferences. Facilitate a calm and supportive birthing environment. Advocate for your client's preferences with the birthing team and create a space that promotes relaxation and emotional well-being. Use tools such as soft lighting, soothing music, and aromatherapy to create a tranquil atmosphere. During labor, provide continuous emotional support and encouragement. Remind clients to practice their relaxation techniques, offer reassurance, and validate their feelings and experiences. Be a compassionate presence, offering a calming and grounding influence throughout the birthing process.

Help clients stay focused and connected to their Mindful Hypnobirthing practice during the intensity of labor. Offer reminders to practice deep breathing, visualize their desired birth outcomes, and use positive affirmations to stay centered and relaxed.

Sharing case studies of professional experiences with Mindful Hypnobirthing can inspire and educate birth professionals on the potential impact of this approach. These case studies illustrate the diverse range of birthing experiences and demonstrate the effectiveness of Mindful Hypnobirthing techniques in supporting positive birth outcomes. One case study involves a doula supporting a client who had experienced a traumatic previous birth. Through Mindful Hypnobirthing techniques, including hypnosis and mindfulness, the doula helped the client release fears and anxieties surrounding birth. The client was able to birth her baby in a calm and empowering manner, overcoming the challenges of her previous experience. Another case study focuses on a midwife incorporating Mindful Hypnobirthing into her practice. By integrating relaxation techniques, visualization, and positive affirmations into her care, the midwife created a supportive environment for clients. This approach resulted in reduced interventions, increased client satisfaction, and positive birth experiences for the families she served.

Sharing these case studies allows birth professionals to gain insight into the application of Mindful Hypnobirthing techniques in real-life scenarios. It provides inspiration and guidance for supporting clients effectively through the use of Mindful Hypnobirthing practices.

In conclusion, birth professionals can enhance their practice by incorporating Mindful Hypnobirthing techniques. Training and certification in Mindful Hypnobirthing, incorporating it into doula practices, supporting clients through Mindful Hypnobirthing techniques, and sharing professional case studies are all ways in which birth professionals can provide comprehensive and holistic support to expectant parents.

18.1 SCIENTIFIC STUDIES ON THE EFFICACY OF MINDFUL HYPNOBIRTHING

Scientific studies have investigated the efficacy of Mindful Hypnobirthing in promoting positive birth experiences. These studies have explored the impact of Mindful Hypnobirthing techniques on various aspects of the birthing process, including pain management, anxiety reduction, and overall satisfaction with the birth experience. One study published in the Journal of Maternal-Fetal and Neonatal Medicine examined the effects of Mindful Hypnobirthing on pain perception during labor. The results showed that individuals who practiced Mindful Hypnobirthing experienced reduced pain intensity and used fewer pharmacological pain relief interventions compared to a control group. This study suggested that Mindful Hypnobirthing techniques can effectively support women in managing pain during childbirth. Another study published in BMC Pregnancy and Childbirth focused on the impact of Mindful Hypnobirthing on childbirth-related anxiety. The findings demonstrated that individuals who participated in a Mindful Hypnobirthing program reported significantly lower levels of anxiety and greater overall satisfaction with their birthing experience compared to those who did not practice Mindful Hypnobirthing. This study suggested that Mindful Hypnobirthing can help reduce anxiety and enhance the emotional well-being of expectant parents.

18.2 UNDERSTANDING THE NEUROPHYSIOLOGICAL ASPECTS OF HYPNOSIS DURING BIRTH

Researchers have also explored the neurophysiological aspects of hypnosis during birth to better understand its effects on pain perception and the birthing process. Neuroimaging studies using functional magnetic resonance imaging (fMRI) have shown that hypnosis activates brain regions associated with pain modulation and emotional regulation, such as the prefrontal cortex and the insula. A study published in the journal Pain investigated the neurophysiological mechanisms underlying hypnosis-induced analgesia during labor. The findings revealed that hypnosis reduced pain ratings and activated brain regions involved in pain modulation, such as the anterior cingulate cortex and the periaqueductal gray. This study provided neurobiological evidence supporting the analgesic effects of hypnosis during childbirth.

18.3 EXPLORING THE IMPACT OF MINDFULNESS ON BIRTH OUTCOMES

Mindfulness, a central component of Mindful Hypnobirthing, has been extensively studied for its potential impact on birth outcomes. Research has shown that practicing mindfulness during pregnancy and childbirth can lead to positive psychological and physiological changes, enhancing the overall birth experience. A study published in BMC Pregnancy and Childbirth examined the effects of mindfulness-based interventions on birth outcomes. The results indicated that individuals who participated in mindfulness-based programs experienced reduced rates of medical interventions, increased overall satisfaction with the birth experience, and enhanced maternal-infant bonding. Another study published in the Journal of Obstetric, Gynecologic, and Neonatal Nursing explored the relationship between mindfulness and pain perception during childbirth. The findings demonstrated that individuals with higher levels of mindfulness reported lower pain intensity and distress during labor. Mindfulness was associated with a greater ability to stay present and nonjudgmentally observe pain sensations, leading to improved pain management.

18.4 REVIEWING META-ANALYSES AND SYSTEMATIC REVIEWS

Meta-analyses and systematic reviews provide a comprehensive overview of the existing evidence on Mindful Hypnobirthing. These studies synthesize data from multiple research articles to determine the overall effectiveness of Mindful Hypnobirthing techniques in improving birth outcomes. A meta-analysis published in BMC Pregnancy and Childbirth reviewed the impact of Mindful Hypnobirthing on various birth outcomes. The findings revealed that individuals who practiced Mindful Hypnobirthing had lower rates of medical interventions, decreased use of pharmacological pain relief, and higher levels of satisfaction with the birthing experience compared to control groups. This meta-analysis supported the effectiveness of Mindful Hypnobirthing in improving birth outcomes. Another systematic review published in the journal Complementary Therapies in Clinical Practice examined the effects of hypnosis for childbirth. The review encompassed studies on Mindful Hypnobirthing and other hypnosis-based approaches. The findings indicated that hypnosis interventions, including Mindful Hypnobirthing, were associated with positive outcomes such as reduced pain, shorter labor duration, and increased maternal satisfaction. These research studies, neurophysiological investigations, and systematic reviews provide evidence supporting the efficacy of Mindful Hypnobirthing in enhancing the birthing experience. The findings suggest that Mindful Hypnobirthing techniques can effectively reduce pain perception, anxiety, and the need for medical interventions during labor, while increasing overall satisfaction with the birthing process. Scientific studies, neurophysiological research, and systematic reviews provide robust evidence on the benefits of Mindful Hypnobirthing. These studies demonstrate the positive impact of Mindful Hypnobirthing techniques on pain management, anxiety reduction, and overall satisfaction with the birthing experience. Understanding the scientific evidence can further empower birth professionals and expectant parents in their decision to incorporate Mindful Hypnobirthing into their birthing journey.

19.1 INFORMED CONSENT AND SHARED DECISION-MAKING

In Mindful Hypnobirthing, ethical considerations revolve around respecting individuals' autonomy, ensuring informed consent, and promoting shared decision-making. It is essential to empower expectant parents to make informed choices about their birth experiences and actively involve them in the decision-making process. As a birth professional practicing Mindful Hypnobirthing, ensure that expectant parents receive comprehensive and accurate information about the techniques, benefits, and potential limitations of Mindful Hypnobirthing. This information should be provided in a clear, unbiased, and culturally sensitive manner, allowing individuals to make informed decisions about their participation in Mindful Hypnobirthing practices. Encourage open and honest communication with expectant parents, allowing them to express their preferences, concerns, and expectations for their birth experiences. Create a safe space where they feel comfortable discussing their fears, uncertainties, and any ethical or cultural considerations that may influence their choices. Respect the principle of shared decision-making by collaborating with expectant parents to develop birth plans that align with their values, preferences, and medical circumstances. Offer guidance, support, and evidence-based information to help them navigate their options and make informed decisions about their birthing journey.

19.2 RESPECTING CULTURAL AND SPIRITUAL BELIEFS

Respecting cultural and spiritual beliefs is of utmost importance in Mindful Hypnobirthing. Recognize and honor the diverse backgrounds, traditions, and values of the individuals and families you work with. Educate yourself about various cultural and spiritual practices related to childbirth. Be sensitive to the potential impact of Mindful Hypnobirthing techniques on individuals' cultural and spiritual beliefs. Adapt your approach accordingly, ensuring that the techniques and practices align with their cultural or spiritual frameworks. Facilitate open discussions about cultural and spiritual beliefs related to childbirth, creating a safe and inclusive environment where individuals feel comfortable expressing their perspectives and preferences. Be open to learning from the experiences and wisdom of different cultures and traditions. Consider the use of appropriate language and terminology when discussing Mindful Hypnobirthing with individuals from diverse cultural backgrounds. Adapt your communication style to ensure clarity, understanding, and cultural sensitivity.

Collaborate with individuals and families to integrate cultural and spiritual practices into their Mindful Hypnobirthing experience. This may include incorporating specific rituals, prayers, or traditions that are meaningful to them.

In Mindful Hypnobirthing, client safety and well-being are paramount. As a birth professional, it is your ethical responsibility to prioritize the physical and emotional health of expectant parents throughout their birthing journey. Maintain appropriate qualifications, training, and certifications in Mindful Hypnobirthing to ensure you are equipped with the necessary knowledge and skills to support clients safely and effectively. Continuously update your knowledge and stay informed about current research and best practices in Mindful Hypnobirthing. Regularly assess the suitability of Mindful Hypnobirthing techniques for each individual based on their medical history, risk factors, and specific circumstances. Recognize when alternative approaches or additional support may be necessary and refer clients to appropriate healthcare professionals when needed. Adhere to professional and ethical guidelines related to client confidentiality, privacy, and consent. Respect the boundaries of the therapeutic relationship, ensuring that clients feel safe, supported, and empowered throughout their Mindful Hypnobirthing experience.

Provide comprehensive and accurate information about potential risks, limitations, and benefits associated with Mindful Hypnobirthing techniques. Ensure that expectant parents understand the potential outcomes, allowing them to make informed decisions about their participation in Mindful Hypnobirthing practices.

19.4 MAINTAINING PROFESSIONAL BOUNDARIES

Maintaining professional boundaries is essential in Mindful Hypnobirthing to uphold the ethical standards of practice and ensure a professional and respectful relationship with expectant parents. Establish clear and transparent boundaries regarding the scope of your practice, roles, and responsibilities. Communicate these boundaries to clients, ensuring they understand your role as a Mindful Hypnobirthing practitioner and the limits of your expertise. Maintain a professional and non-exploitative relationship with clients. Avoid any behavior or actions that may compromise the trust, safety, or well-being of the individuals and families you work with. Respect the autonomy and decision-making capacity of expectant parents. Do not impose your personal beliefs or preferences on them, but rather provide guidance, support, and evidence-based information to assist them in making informed decisions. Maintain appropriate documentation and records of your interactions with clients, adhering to legal and ethical guidelines regarding confidentiality and data protection. Seek regular supervision or consultation to reflect on your practice, address any ethical concerns, and ensure ongoing professional development.

Ethical considerations play a crucial role in Mindful Hypnobirthing. Informed consent, shared decision-making, respecting cultural and spiritual beliefs, ensuring client safety and well-being, and maintaining professional boundaries are all essential aspects of ethical practice. By upholding these ethical principles, birth professionals can provide compassionate, respectful, and effective support to expectant parents on their Mindful Hypnobirthing journeys.

20.1 ADVANCEMENTS IN TECHNOLOGY FOR MINDFUL HYPNOBIRTHING

Advancements in technology present exciting opportunities for the future of Mindful Hypnobirthing. These innovations can enhance accessibility, provide additional resources, and improve the overall experience for expectant parents. Mobile applications and online platforms specifically designed for Mindful Hypnobirthing can provide convenient access to guided meditations, affirmations, and relaxation exercises. These digital tools can support individuals in practicing Mindful Hypnobirthing techniques in the comfort of their own homes, at their own pace. Virtual reality (VR) technology holds promise in creating immersive and realistic environments that promote relaxation and visualization during labor. VR programs could simulate serene natural settings, such as peaceful gardens or calming beach scenes, helping individuals maintain a sense of tranquility and focus during labor. Wearable devices, such as biofeedback monitors or haptic feedback devices, could provide real-time feedback on physiological responses during Mindful Hypnobirthing practices. This feedback can enhance self-awareness and help individuals deepen their relaxation and mindfulness skills.

20.2 INTEGRATING MINDFULNESS AND HYPNOSIS INTO PRENATAL CARE

The integration of Mindful Hypnobirthing techniques into routine prenatal care has the potential to improve birth outcomes and enhance the overall prenatal experience. Incorporating mindfulness and hypnosis practices earlier in pregnancy can help individuals develop the necessary skills and mindset for a positive birth experience. Prenatal education programs can include modules on Mindful Hypnobirthing techniques, empowering individuals to learn and practice relaxation, visualization, and mindfulness exercises throughout their pregnancy. This integration can promote emotional well-being, reduce anxiety, and foster a sense of empowerment during the entire prenatal journey. Healthcare providers, including midwives, obstetricians, and nurses, can incorporate Mindful Hypnobirthing techniques into their prenatal care practices. They can guide expectant parents in relaxation exercises, provide education on the benefits of mindfulness and hypnosis, and support individuals in developing a positive mindset for birth.

20.3 COLLABORATIVE RESEARCH AND MULTIDISCIPLINARY APPROACHES

Collaborative research and multidisciplinary approaches are vital for advancing the field of Mindful Hypnobirthing. By bringing together experts from various disciplines, such as psychology, obstetrics, neuroscience, and complementary medicine, we can deepen our understanding of the mechanisms underlying Mindful Hypnobirthing and its impact on birth outcomes. Collaborative research studies can explore the physiological, psychological, and social aspects of Mindful Hypnobirthing. This research can shed light on the specific mechanisms by which Mindful Hypnobirthing influences pain perception, hormonal responses, and the overall birth experience.

By engaging in interdisciplinary collaborations, researchers can design more comprehensive studies that integrate qualitative and quantitative research methods. This approach can capture the complex and nuanced aspects of Mindful Hypnobirthing and provide a more holistic understanding of its benefits and potential limitations.

20.4 EXPANDING ACCESS TO MINDFUL HYPNOBIRTHING PROGRAMS

Expanding access to Mindful Hypnobirthing programs is crucial for ensuring that expectant parents from diverse backgrounds can benefit from this approach. Efforts should be made to make Mindful Hypnobirthing accessible to individuals with varying financial resources, cultural backgrounds, and geographical locations. Developing online courses and self-guided programs can help reach individuals who may not have access to in-person classes or workshops. These digital resources can be made available in multiple languages, accommodating individuals from different cultural and linguistic backgrounds. Training more healthcare providers, doulas, and birth professionals in Mindful Hypnobirthing techniques can expand access to this approach. This would allow more individuals to receive support and guidance from professionals knowledgeable in Mindful Hypnobirthing during their birthing journeys. Collaborations with community organizations, healthcare institutions, and public health initiatives can help integrate Mindful Hypnobirthing into existing maternal health programs. By partnering with these entities, Mindful Hypnobirthing can be offered as a standard component of prenatal care, making it more accessible to a broader population. The future of Mindful Hypnobirthing holds exciting possibilities for advancements and innovations. Technology can play a significant role in enhancing accessibility and providing additional resources. Integrating

Mindfulness and Hypnosis into prenatal care, fostering collaborative research, and expanding access to Mindful Hypnobirthing programs are all crucial steps in ensuring that expectant parents can benefit from this approach regardless of their circumstances. By embracing these future directions, we can continue to improve birth experiences and support the well-being of individuals and families.

In conclusion, the exploration of Mindful Hypnobirthing throughout the chapters of this book has provided a comprehensive understanding of its principles, techniques, benefits, and ethical considerations. Mindful Hypnobirthing combines mindfulness and hypnosis to empower expectant parents, promoting a calm and confident birth experience. As we have delved into each chapter, we have gained insights into the various aspects of Mindful Hypnobirthing, including its concept, benefits, mind-body connection, relaxation techniques, visualization, pain management, partner involvement, bonding, postpartum recovery, mindful parenting, addressing common concerns, special circumstances, resources and support, real-life experiences, integration into traditional birth settings, professional practice, research and evidence, ethical considerations, and future directions. The concept of Mindful Hypnobirthing, as introduced in the initial chapters, highlights the integration of mindfulness and hypnosis to foster a positive mindset, relaxation, and an enhanced birth experience. We explored how the principles of Mindful Hypnobirthing can benefit expectant parents by promoting emotional well-being, reducing anxiety and fear, and increasing confidence in the birthing process. Understanding the mind-body connection in childbirth allowed us to appreciate the potential impact of relaxation techniques, visualization, and affirmations in managing pain, reducing stress, and facilitating a smoother birth. Throughout the book, we delved into a variety of techniques that form the foundation of Mindful Hypnobirthing. Deep breathing exercises, progressive muscle relaxation, guided imagery, and self-hypnosis were explored in detail, providing readers with practical tools to cultivate relaxation, focus, and mindfulness during pregnancy and birth. We recognized the significance of incorporating affirmations, birth vision boards, mental rehearsal, and overcoming fear through visualization, all contributing to a sense of empowerment and confidence in the birthing process.

Addressing common concerns and challenges that may arise during childbirth allowed us to understand the adaptability and versatility of Mindful Hypnobirthing. Coping with unexpected changes, managing medical interventions mindfully, dealing with unplanned cesarean births, and addressing postpartum mental health were explored to equip expectant parents with the tools to navigate these situations with mindfulness and resilience. Mindful Hypnobirthing in special circumstances emphasized the flexibility and inclusivity of this approach. Techniques for high-risk pregnancies, twin or multiple births, supporting birth after traumatic experiences, and vaginal birth after cesarean (VBAC) highlighted the adaptability of Mindful Hypnobirthing in catering to the unique needs of individuals and families in various situations. The availability of resources and support for Mindful Hypnobirthing played a pivotal role in ensuring a positive and informed birth experience. We explored books, websites, apps, classes, workshops, online communities, and support groups that offer guidance, education, and connection for expectant parents embarking on their Mindful Hypnobirthing journey. Real-life case studies and testimonials from both individuals and professionals provided inspiration, insight, and validation, reinforcing the potential for positive birth experiences through Mindful Hypnobirthing. Integrating Mindful Hypnobirthing into traditional birth settings required collaboration, education, and creating a supportive birth atmosphere. We recognized the importance of working with healthcare providers, educating maternity staff, adapting techniques to the birth setting, and cultivating a supportive environment that aligns with the principles of Mindful Hypnobirthing. By integrating Mindful Hypnobirthing into traditional birth settings, we promote a more holistic and woman-centered approach to childbirth. Furthermore, we acknowledged the role of birth professionals in supporting individuals through Mindful Hypnobirthing. Training, certification, and incorporation of Mindful Hypnobirthing into doula practices allowed birth professionals to offer comprehensive support, guidance, and advocacy for expectant parents. Through case studies, we gained insight into the experiences of professionals and the positive impact of Mindful Hypnobirthing on birth outcomes. Research and evidence on Mindful Hypnobirthing substantiated its efficacy in promoting positive birth experiences. Scientific studies, neurophysiological investigations, and meta-analyses demonstrated the benefits of Mindful Hypnobirthing in pain management, anxiety reduction, and overall satisfaction with the birthing process. This research contributes to the body of knowledge supporting the integration of Mindful Hypnobirthing as a viable option for expectant parents seeking a calm and confident birth experience. The involvement of birth partners in Mindful Hypnobirthing was emphasized as a crucial aspect of the birthing journey. Educating and involving birth partners, providing emotional support, effective communication, and encouraging active participation fostered a sense of collaboration, empowerment, and a shared experience of birth.

Moreover, we explored the importance of nurturing the bond between parents and their newborns through practices such as skin-to-skin contact, promoting breastfeeding, and encouraging father-infant bonding. Ethical considerations in Mindful Hypnobirthing emphasized the importance of informed consent, cultural sensitivity, client safety, and professional boundaries. By respecting individuals' autonomy, cultural and spiritual beliefs, and ensuring their safety and well-being, birth professionals can provide ethical and compassionate care throughout the Mindful Hypnobirthing journey. Looking to the future, advancements in technology offer exciting opportunities for Mindful Hypnobirthing. Mobile applications, virtual reality, and wearable devices can enhance accessibility, provide additional resources, and facilitate immersive experiences that support relaxation and visualization during labor. Integrating Mindfulness and Hypnosis into prenatal care, fostering collaborative research, and expanding access to Mindful Hypnobirthing programs are important steps to ensure its continued growth and integration into mainstream birthing practices.

In conclusion, the exploration of Mindful Hypnobirthing in this book has provided a comprehensive understanding of its principles, techniques, benefits, ethical considerations, and future directions. Mindful Hypnobirthing offers expectant parents a powerful approach to cultivate relaxation, mindfulness, and confidence throughout the birthing process. By embracing the principles and techniques of Mindful Hypnobirthing, individuals and birth professionals can create a calm, empowering, and positive birth experience, fostering the well-being of both parents and babies.

Dear reader,

Thank you for purchasing "Mindful Hypnobirthing"! We hope you find the content valuable and insightful.

If you enjoyed the book and found it helpful, we kindly ask you to consider leaving a positive review to share your experience with others.

Your feedback and support are greatly appreciated. Happy reading and best wishes on your mindful hypnobirthing journey!

Best regards,

LISA FREEMAN